AIR FRYER KETO COOKBOOK

The Ultimate Keto Air Fryer Cookbook for Burn Fat With Quick and and Easy Keto Recipes.

Boost your Brain Health and Lose Weight.

KetonUSA

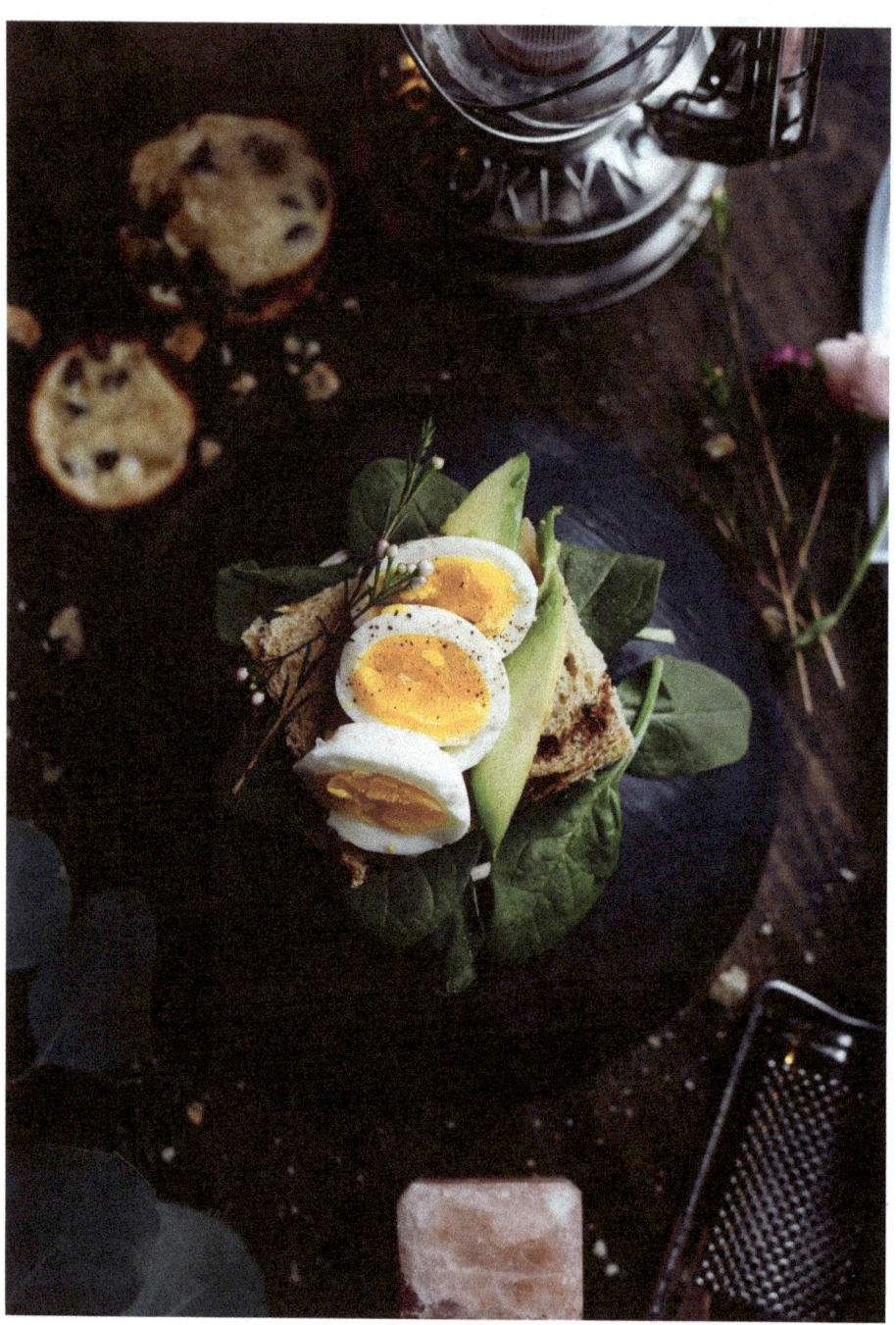

© Copyright 2021 by KetonUSA- All rights reserved. The following Book is reproduced below with the goal of providing information that is as accurate and reliable as possible. Regardless, purchasing this Book can be seen as consent to the fact that both the publisher and the author of this book are in no way experts on the topics discussed within and that any recommendations or suggestions that are made herein are for entertainment purposes only. Professionals should be consulted as needed prior to undertaking any of the action endorsed herein.

This declaration is deemed fair and valid by both the American Bar Association and the Committee of Publishers Association and is legally binding throughout the United States.

Furthermore, the transmission, duplication, or reproduction of any of the following work including specific information will be considered an illegal act irrespective of if it is done electronically or in print. This extends to creating a secondary or tertiary copy of the work or a recorded copy and is only allowed with the express written consent from the Publisher. All additional right reserved.

The information in the following pages is broadly considered a truthful and accurate account of facts and as such, any inattention, use, or misuse of the information in question by the reader will render any resulting actions solely under their purview. There are no scenarios in which the publisher or the original author of this work can be in any fashion deemed liable for any hardship or damages that may befall them after undertaking information described herein.

Additionally, the information in the following pages is intended only for informational purposes and should thus be thought of as universal. As befitting its nature, it is presented without assurance regarding its prolonged validity or interim quality. Trademarks that are mentioned are done without written consent and can in no way be considered an endorsement from the trademark holder.

Table of Contents

CRUNCHY GRANOLA 6
JALAPENO POPPER EGG CUPS 9
CRISPY SOUTHWESTERN HAM EGG CUPS 11
BUFFALO EGG CUPS 13
VEGGIE FRITTATA 15
PUMPKIN SPICE MUFFINS 17
QUICK AND EASY BACON STRIPS 20
BANANA NUT CAKE 22
LEMON POPPY SEED CAKE 25
PANCAKE CAKE 28
BACON, EGG, AND CHEESE ROLL UPS 31
CHEESY CAULIFLOWER HASH BROWNS 34
BREAKFAST STUFFED POBLANO 36
AIR FRYER "HARD-BOILED" EGGS 39
SCRAMBLED EGGS 41
LOADED CAULIFLOWER BREAKFAST BAKE 44
CINNAMON ROLL STICKS 46
BREAKFAST CALZONE 49
CAULIFLOWER AVOCADO TOAST 53
SAUSAGE AND CHEESE BALLS 55
CHEESY BELL PEPPER EGGS 58
SPAGHETTI SQUASH FRITTERS 60
BREAKFAST EGG BOWLS 62
DELICIOUS BREAKFAST SOUFFLÉ PREPARATION 64
AIR FRIED SANDWICH 66
RUSTIC BREAKFAST PREPARATION 67
EGG MUFFINS PREPARATION 69
POLENTA BITES 71
DELICIOUS BREAKFAST POTATOES 73
TASTY CINNAMON TOAST 75
DELICIOUS POTATO HASH 77
SWEET BREAKFAST CASSEROLE 78
EGGS CASSEROLE 80
SAUSAGE, EGGS AND CHEESE MIX 81
CHEESE AIR FRIED BAKE 83
BISCUITS CASSEROLE 84
TURKEY BURRITO 86
TOFU SCRAMBLE 88
OATMEAL CASSEROLE 90
HAM BREAKFAST 92

Tomato and Bacon Breakfast	94
Tasty Hash	96
Creamy Hash Browns	97
Blackberry French Toast	99
Smoked Sausage Breakfast Mix	101
Delicious Potato Frittata	103
Asparagus Frittata	105
Special Corn Flakes Breakfast Casserole	106
Ham Breakfast Pie	108
Breakfast Veggie Mix	109

Crunchy Granola

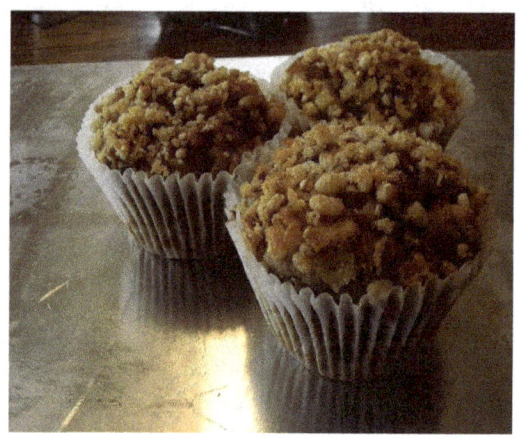

Missing the crunch of cereal in the morning? This recipe saves the day in a simple way because making it is as easy as mixing all the ingredients together and popping it in your air fryer! Once the granola is done, you can enjoy it in a bowl of unsweetened nut milk or on top of a low-carb, full-fat yogurt!

- HandsOn Time: 10 minutes
- Cook Time: 5 minutes

Serves 6

- 2 cups pecans, chopped
  - 1 cup unsweetened coconut flakes

- 1 cup almond slivers
- 1/3 cup sunflower seeds
- 1/4 cup golden flaxseed
- 1/4 cup low-carb, sugar- free chocolate chips
- 1/4 cup granular erythritol
- 2 tablespoons unsalted butter
- 1 teaspoon ground cinnamon

Directions

- ✓ In a large bowl, mix all ingredients.
- ✓ Place the mixture into a 4-cup round baking dish. Place dish into the air fryer basket.
- ✓ Adjust the temperature to 320°F and set the timer for 5 minutes.
- ✓ Allow to cool completely before serving.

PER SERVING

Calories: 617 Protein: 10.9 G Fiber: 11.2 G
Net Carbohydrates: 6.5 G Sugar Alcohol: 14.7 G

Fat: 55.8 G Sodium: 5 Mg Carbohydrates: 32.4 G Sugar: 2.7 G

WAYS TO ENJOY

You can enjoy this granola with a bowl of unsweetened almond milk, or make it a parfait by mixing up a keto "faux-gurt" made simply of V2 cup sour cream, 1 tablespoon heavy cream, and 1 tablespoon of your favorite low-carb sweetener!

Jalapeno Popper Egg Cups

The savory goodness of this classic appetizer has finally come to breakfast! Spice up your morning with eggs that pack a serious punch and crunch! Be sure to make enough for second helpings . . . you'll be glad you did!

- HandsOn Time: 10 minutes
- Cook Time: 10 minutes

Serves 2

- 4 large eggs
- 1/4 cup chopped pickled jalapenos 2 ounces full-fat cream cheese
- 1/2 cup shredded sharp Cheddar cheese

Directions

✓ In a medium bowl, beat the eggs, then pour into four silicone muffin cups.

✓ In a large microwave-safe bowl, place jalapenos, cream cheese, and Cheddar. Microwave for 30 seconds and stir.

✓ Take a spoonful, approximately ¼ of the mixture, and place it in the center of one of the egg cups. Repeat with remaining mixture.

✓ Place egg cups into the air fryer basket.

✓ Adjust the temperature to 320°F and set the timer for 10 minutes. Serve warm.

PER SERVING

Calories: 354

Protein: 21.0 G Fiber: 0.2 G

Net Carbohydrates: 2.1 G Fat: 25.3 G

Sodium: 601 Mg Carbohydrates: 2.3 G Sugar: 1.4 G

Crispy Southwestern Ham Egg Cups

This recipe, cooked right in the cups lined with delicious ham, will start your day with a burst of creamy, subtly spicy Southwestern flavor. The sour cream in the dish helps cut the spice and adds fat to your meal that helps keep you full!

- HandsOn Time: 5 minutes
- Cook Time: 12 minutes

Serves 2

- 4 (1-ounce) slices deli ham 4 large eggs
- 2 tablespoons full-fat sour cream
- 1/4 cup diced green bell pepper 2 tablespoons diced red bell pepper 2 tablespoons diced white onion 1/2 cup shredded medium Cheddar cheese

Directions

✓ Place one slice of ham on the bottom of four baking cups.
✓ In a large bowl, whisk eggs with sour cream. Stir in green pepper, red pepper, and onion.

- ✓ Pour the egg mixture into ham-lined baking cups.
- ✓ Top with Cheddar. Place cups into the air fryer basket.
- ✓ Adjust the temperature to 320°F and set the timer for 12 minutes or until the tops are browned.
- ✓ Serve warm.

PER SERVING

Calories: 382

Protein: 29.4 G Fiber: 1.4 G

Net Carbohydrates: 4.6 G Fat: 23.6 G

Sodium: 977 Mg Carbohydrates: 6.0 G Sugar: 2.1 G

Buffalo Egg Cups

Looking for a great way to take your morning eggs to the next level while packing in an extra boost of protein? These Buffalo Egg Cups are your answer. The spicy buffalo sauce will satisfy your palate, and the eggs' fat and protein will work together to keep you full!

- HandsOn Time: 10 minutes
- Cook Time: 15 minutes

Serves 2

- 4 large eggs
- 2 ounces full-fat cream cheese
- 2 tablespoons buffalo sauce
- 1/2 cup shredded sharp Cheddar cheese

Directions

✓ Crack eggs into two (4") ramekins.

✓ In a small microwave-safe bowl, mix cream cheese, buffalo sauce, and Cheddar.

✓ Microwave for 20 seconds and then stir.

✓ Place a spoonful into each ramekin on top of the eggs.

✓ Place ramekins into the air fryer basket. Adjust the temperature to 320°F and set the timer for 15 minutes. Serve warm.

PER SERVING

Calories: 354
Protein: 21.0 G Fiber: 0.0 G
Net Carbohydrates: 2.3 G Fat: 22.3 G
Sodium: 886 Mg Carbohydrates: 2.3 G Sugar: 1.4 G

Veggie Frittata

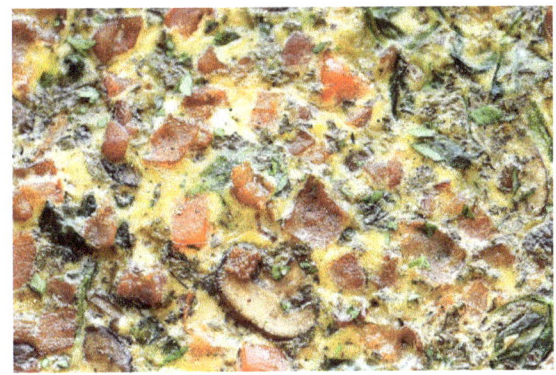

Want to get your day started with a nutritious and filling boost? This breakfast is just what you need to help you get your daily veggies in early! Of course vegetables are packed with nutrients to help keep you healthy and strong, but it's important to keep an eye on the carb counts because vegetables have a huge range.

- HandsOn Time: 15 minutes
- Cook Time: 12 minutes

Serves 4

- 6 large eggs
- 1/4 cup heavy whipping cream

- 1/2 cup chopped broccoli
- 1/4 cup chopped yellow onion
- 1/4 cup chopped green bell pepper

Directions

✓ In a large bowl, whisk eggs and heavy whipping cream.

✓ Mix in broccoli, onion, and bell pepper.

✓ Pour into a 6" round oven-safe baking dish.

✓ Place baking dish into the air fryer basket.

✓ Adjust the temperature to 350°F and set the timer for 12 minutes.

✓ Eggs should be firm and cooked fully when the frittata is done. Serve warm.

PER SERVING

Calories: 168
Protein: 10.2 G Fiber: 0.6 G
Net Carbohydrates: 2.5 G Fat: 11.8 G
Sodium: 116 Mg Carbohydrates: 3.1 G Sugar: 1.5 G

Pumpkin Spice Muffins

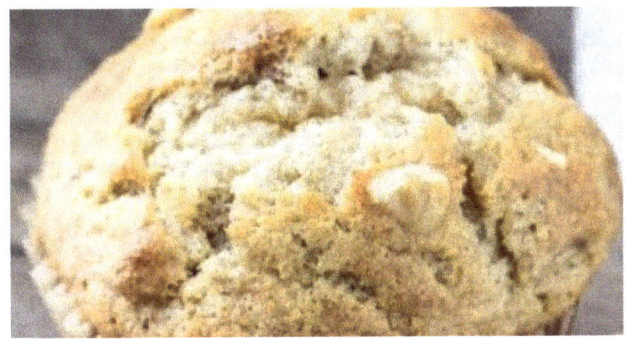

Who doesn't love the taste of pumpkin on a crisp autumn morning? For most people, pumpkin and fall go hand in hand, and this recipe will be a staple in your breakfast rotation all season long!

- HandsOn Time: 10 minutes

- Cook Time: 15 minutes

Serves 6

- 1 cup blanched finely ground almond flour

- 1/2 cup granular erythritol

- 1/2 teaspoon baking powder

- 1/4 cup unsalted butter, softened

- 1/4 cup pure pumpkin puree
- 1/2 teaspoon ground cinnamon
- 1/4 teaspoon ground nutmeg
- 1 teaspoon vanilla extract
- 2 large eggs

Directions

✓ In a large bowl, mix almond flour, erythritol, baking powder, butter, pumpkin puree, cinnamon, nutmeg, and vanilla. Gently stir in eggs.

✓ Evenly pour the batter into six silicone muffin cups. Place muffin cups into the air fryer basket, working in batches if necessary.

✓ Adjust the temperature to 300°F and set the timer for 15 minutes.

✓ When completely cooked, a toothpick inserted in center will come out mostly clean. Serve warm.

PER SERVING

Calories: 205 Protein: 6.3 G Fiber: 2.4 G Net Carbohydrates Sodium: 65 Mg Carbohydrates: 17.4 G Sugar

Make sure you use regular pumpkin puree instead of pumpkin pie puree! It can be tricky because they're usually right next to each other on store shelves, but the latter has added carbs and sugar that you definitely don't need for this flavorful treat!

Quick and Easy Bacon Strips

What's better than perfectly crisped bacon in the morning? Gone are the days of cautiously standing over a hot pan while grease splatters at you. With your air fryer, you're just minutes away from delicious strips of evenly cooked bacon every time!

- HandsOn Time: 5 minutes
- Cook Time: 12 minutes

Serves 4

- 8 slices sugar-free bacon

Directions

✓ Place bacon strips into the air fryer basket.
✓ Adjust the temperature to 400°F and set the timer for 12 minutes.
✓ After 6 minutes, flip bacon and continue cooking time. Serve warm.

PER SERVING

Calories: 88 Protein: 5.8 G Fiber: 0.0 G Net Carbohydrates: 0.2 G Fat: 6.2 G Sodium: 355 Mg Carbohydrates: 0.2 G Sugar: 0.0 G

Banana Nut Cake

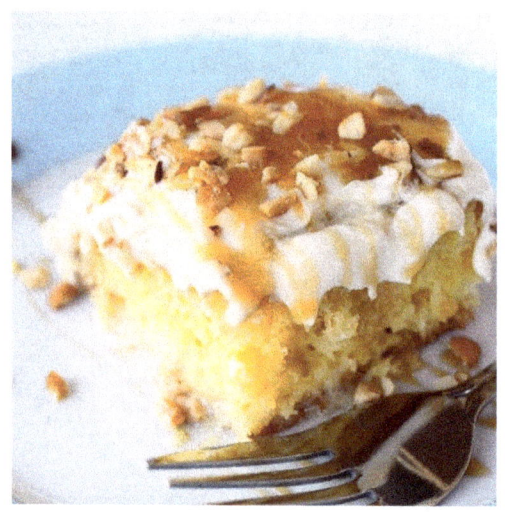

Even though bananas aren't a great option for keto because of high carb count, you can still enjoy banana nut cake by employing the help of the very low-carb banana extract. You can customize these muffins to your liking by swapping out the walnuts for your favorite nut.

- HandsOn Time: 15 minutes
- Cook Time: 25 minutes

Serves 6

- 1 cup blanched finely ground almond flour

- 1/2 cup powdered erythritol
- 2 tablespoons ground golden flaxseed
- 2 teaspoons baking powder
- 1/2 teaspoon ground cinnamon
- 1/4 cup unsalted butter, melted
- 2 1/2 teaspoons banana extract
- 1 teaspoon vanilla extract
- 1/4 cup full-fat sour cream
- 2 large eggs
- 1/4 cup chopped walnuts

Directions

✓ In a large bowl, mix almond flour, erythritol, flaxseed, baking powder, and cinnamon.

✓ Stir in butter, banana extract, vanilla extract, and sour cream.

✓ Add eggs to the mixture and gently stir until fully combined. Stir in the walnuts. ✓ ✓ Pour into 6" nonstick cake pan and place into the air fryer basket.

✓ Adjust the temperature to 300°F and set the timer for 25 minutes.

✓ Cake will be golden and a toothpick inserted in center will come out clean when fully cooked. Allow to fully cool to avoid crumbling.

PER SERVING

Calories: 263 Protein: 7.6 G Fiber: 3.1 G
Net Carbohydrates: 3.3 G Sugar Alcohol: 12.0 G Fat: 23.6 G
Sodium: 192 Mg Carbohydrates: 18.4 G Sugar: 1.3 G

WHY NOT REAL BANANAS?

- One medium banana has about 24 grams of net carbohydrates. That's more than you would probably eat in a whole day!

- Banana extract is an excellent replacement that can be found in your local grocery store.

Lemon Poppy Seed Cake

You can set this cake cooking when you get up in the morning, hop in the shower, and return to a moist and delicious low-carb treat that will be hard to put down! It's a great way to get your day started with a smile on your face!

- HandsOn Time: 10 minutes
- Cook Time: 14 minutes

Serves 6

- 1 cup b lanched finely ground almond flour
- 1/2 cup powdered erythritol
- 1/2 teaspoon baking powder
- 1/4 cup unsalted butter,
- melted 1/4 cup unsweetened almond milk
- 2 large eggs
- 1 teaspoon vanilla extract
- 1 medium lemon
- 1 teaspoon poppy seeds

Directions

✓ In a large bowl, mix almond flour, erythritol, baking powder, butter, almond milk, eggs, and vanilla.

✓ Slice the lemon in half and squeeze the juice into a small bowl, then add to the batter.

✓ Using a fine grater, zest the lemon and add 1 tablespoon zest to the batter and stir.

✓ Add poppy seeds to batter.

✓ Pour batter into nonstick 6" round cake pan. Place pan into the air fryer basket.

✓ Adjust the temperature to 300°F and set the timer for 14 minutes.

✓ When fully cooked, a toothpick inserted in center will come out mostly clean. The cake will finish cooking and firm up as it cools. Serve at room temperature.

PER SERVING

Calories: 204 Protein: 6.3 G Fiber: 2.4 G
Net Carbohydrates: 2.5 G Sugar Alcohol: 12.0 G Fat: 18.2 G Sodium: 72 Mg Carbohydrates: 16.9 G Sugar: 0.9 G

Pancake Cake

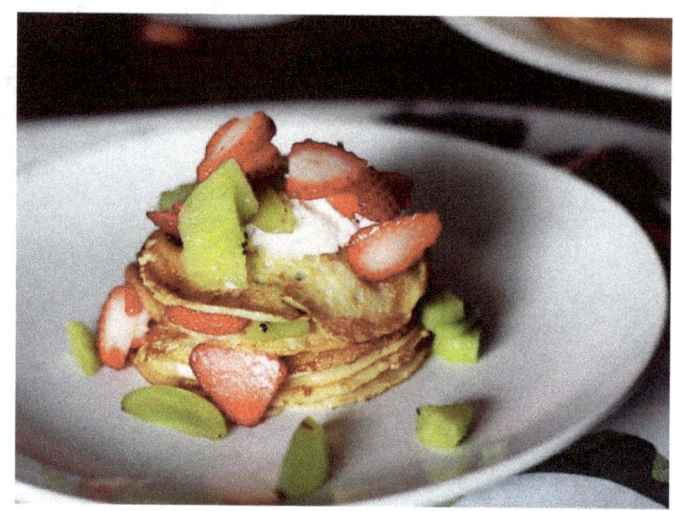

This bakes up quick for a fluffy and delicious breakfast for the whole family. It's a treat that the kids will love, and you'll love how simple it is to make! For added fun, you can throw in a handful of low-carb chocolate chips! Serve this with low-carb syrup or sugar-free whipped cream and low- carb berries such as strawberries or blackberries.

- HandsOn Time: 10 minutes
- Cook Time: 7 minutes

Serves 4

- 1/2 cup blanched finely ground almond flour
- 1/4 cup powdered erythritol
- 1/2 teaspoon baking powder
- 2 tablespoons unsalted butter,
- softened 1 large egg
- 1/2 teaspoon unflavored gelatin
- 1/2 teaspoon vanilla extract
- 1/2 teaspoon ground cinnamon

Directions

✓ In a large bowl, mix almond flour, erythritol, and baking powder. Add butter, egg, gelatin, vanilla, and cinnamon. Pour into 6" round baking pan.

✓ Place pan into the air fryer basket.

✓ Adjust the temperature to 300°F and set the timer for 7 minutes.

✓ When the cake is completely cooked, a toothpick will come out clean. Cut cake into four and serve.

PER SERVING

Calories: 153 Protein: 5.4 G Fiber: 1.7 G Net Carbohydrates Sodium: 80 Mg Carbohydrates: 12.6 G Sugar

Bacon, Egg, and Cheese Roll Ups

This is the tastiest spin on a breakfast burrito you've ever tried! With all of the carbs in a regular tortilla, why not just replace the wrap altogether with crispy and savory bacon? Load your burrito up with all the goods, and pick it up just like the classic version!

- HandsOn Time: 15 minutes
- Cook Time: 15 minutes

Serves 4

- 2 tablespoons unsalted butter
- 1/4 cup chopped onion
- 1/2 medium green bell pepper, seeded and chopped
- 6 large eggs
- 12 slices sugar-free bacon
- 1 cup shredded sharp Cheddar cheese
- 1/2 cup mild salsa, for dipping

Directions

✓ In a medium skillet over medium heat, melt butter.

✓ Add onion and pepper to the skillet and saute until fragrant and onions are translucent, about 3 minutes.

✓ Whisk eggs in a small bowl and pour into skillet.

✓ Scramble eggs with onions and peppers until fluffy and fully cooked, about 5 minutes. Remove from heat and set aside.

✓ On work surface, place three slices of bacon side by side, overlapping about V4".

✓ Place V4 cup scrambled eggs in a heap on the side closest to you and sprinkle V4 cup cheese on top of the eggs.

✓ Tightly roll the bacon around the eggs and secure the seam with a toothpick if necessary.

✓ Place each roll into the air fryer basket.

✓ Adjust the temperature to 350°F and set the timer for 15 minutes. Rotate the rolls halfway through the cooking time.

✓ Bacon will be brown and crispy when completely cooked. Serve immediately with salsa for dipping.

PER SERVING

Calories: 460 Protein: 28.2 G Fiber: 0.8 G Net Carbohydrates: 5.3 G Fat: 31.7 G Sodium: 1,100 Mg Carbohydrates: 6.1 G Sugar: 3.1 G

MAKE IT YOUR OWN!

- Customize this dish with your favorite egg add-ins! Chopped onions, mushrooms, or spinach are all great low-carb options. If you're extra hungry, adding some cooked crumbled breakfast sausage will make this even more filling!

Cheesy Cauliflower Hash Browns

High-carb potatoes aren't a good option for keto, cauliflower makes a great nutrient-dense, low-carb substitute for hash browns. And with the help of your air fryer, you can get them perfectly crispy in no time at all! The cheese in this recipe helps bind the cauliflower together and adds an irresistible flavor that your whole family will love!

- HandsOn Time: 20 minutes

- Cook Time: 12 minutes

Serves 4

- 1 (12-ounce) steamer bag cauliflower
- 1 large egg
- 1 cup shredded sharp Cheddar cheese

   Directions

✓ Place bag in microwave and cook according to package instructions. Allow to cool completely and put cauliflower into a cheesecloth or kitchen towel and squeeze to remove excess moisture.

✓ Mash cauliflower with a fork and add egg and cheese.

✓ Cut a piece of parchment to fit your air fryer basket. Take ¼ of the mixture and form it into a hash brown patty shape.

✓ Place it onto the parchment and into the air fryer basket, working in batches if necessary.

✓ Adjust the temperature to 400°F and set the timer for 12 minutes.

Flip the hash browns halfway through the cooking time. When completely cooked, they will be golden brown. Serve immediately.

PER SERVING

Calories: 153

Protein: 10.0 G Fiber: 1.7 G Net Carbohydrates: 3.0 G Fat: 9.5 G Sodium: 225 Mg Carbohydrates: 4.7 G Sugar: 1.8 G

Breakfast Stuffed Poblano

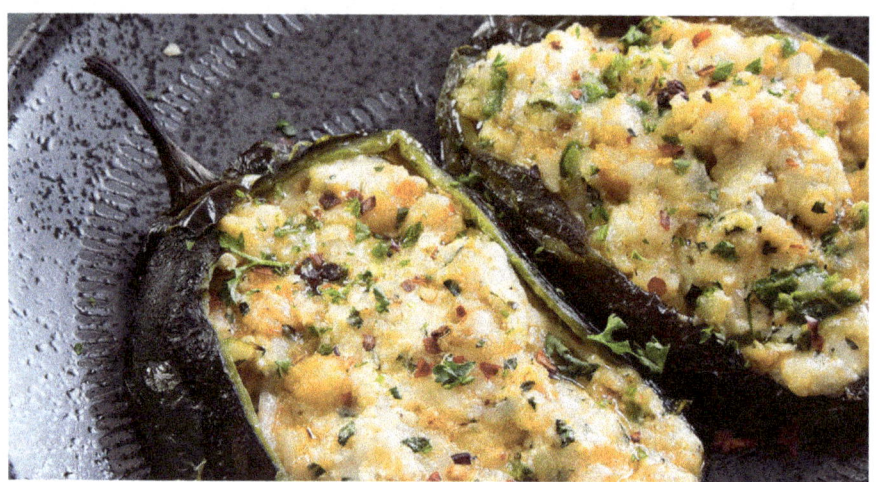

Get ready for a brand-new breakfast in your weekly rotation. This morning spin on jalapeno poppers will give you the kick you need to start your day. Crisped perfectly in your air fryer, this will also become a favorite for those "breakfast for dinner" nights!

- HandsOn Time: 15 minutes

- Cook Time: 15 minutes

Serves 4

- 1/2 pound spicy ground pork breakfast sausage
- 4 large eggs
- 4 ounces full-fat cream cheese, softened

- 1/4 cup canned diced tomatoes and green chiles,

- drained 4 large poblano peppers

- 8 tablespoons shredded pepper jack cheese

- 1/2 cup full-fat sour cream

Directions

✓ In a medium skillet over medium heat, crumble and brown the ground sausage until no pink remains.

✓ Remove sausage and drain the fat from the pan.

✓ Crack eggs into the pan, scramble, and cook until no longer runny.

✓ Place cooked sausage in a large bowl and fold in cream cheese. Mix in diced tomatoes and chiles. Gently fold in eggs.

✓ Cut a 4"-5" slit in the top of each poblano, removing the seeds and white membrane with a small knife.

✓ Separate the filling into four servings and spoon carefully into each pepper. Top each with 2 tablespoons pepper jack cheese.

✓ Place each pepper into the air fryer basket.

✓ Adjust the temperature to 350°F and set the for 15 minutes.

✓ Peppers will be soft and cheese will be browned when ready. Serve immediately with sour cream on top.

PER SERVING

Calories: 489 Protein: 22.8 G Fiber: 3.8 G

Net Carbohydrates: 8.8 G Fat: 35.6 G Sodium: 746 Mg

Carbohydrates: 12.6 G Sugar: 2.9 G

Air Fryer "Hard-Boiled" Eggs

Yes, it is possible to "hard-boil" whole eggs in your air fryer! This method may seem a bit out of the ordinary, but it's a great way to achieve the same results you're used to without having to boil a pot of water on the stove! This is the perfect way to prepare several grab-and-go snacks to support your ketogenic lifestyle.

• HandsOn Time: 2 minutes • Cook Time: 18 minutes Serves 4

- 4 large eggs
- 1 cup water

Directions

✓ Place eggs into a 4-cup round baking-safe dish and pour water over eggs. Place dish into the air fryer basket.

✓ Adjust the temperature to 300°F and set the timer for 18 minutes.

✓ Store cooked eggs in the refrigerator until ready to use or peel and eat warm.

PER SERVING

Calories: 77 Protein: 6.3 G Fiber: 0.0 G Net Carbohydrates: 0.6 G Fat: 4.4 G Sodium: 62 Mg Carbohydrates: 0.6 G Sugar: 0.6 G

Scrambled Eggs

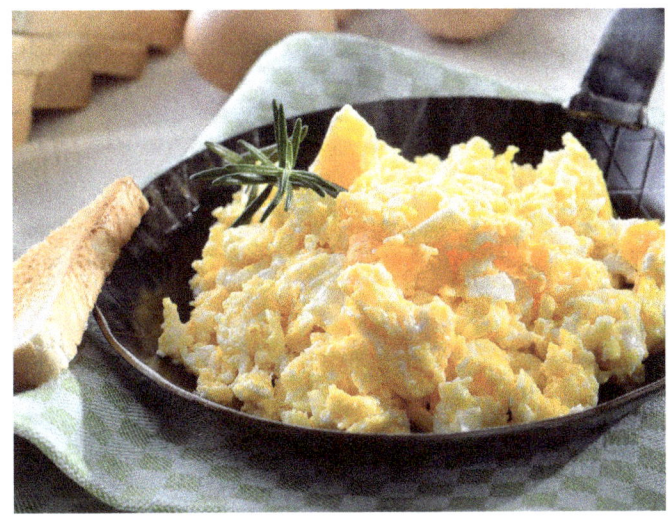

Sometimes you just don't want to turn on your stove, or you don't have access to it for whatever reason. When you're in a pinch, you can still get classic moist Scrambled Eggs from your air fryer!

• HandsOn Time: 5 minutes • Cook Time: 15 minutes Serves 2

- 4 large eggs

- 2 tablespoons unsalted butter,

- Melted 1/2 cup shredded sharp Cheddar cheese

Directions

✓ Crack eggs into 2-cup round baking dish and whisk. Place dish into the air fryer basket.

✓ Adjust the temperature to 400°F and set the timer for 10 minutes.

✓ After 5 minutes, stir the eggs and add the butter and cheese. Let cook 3 more minutes and stir again.

✓ Allow eggs to finish cooking an additional 2 minutes or remove if they are to your desired liking.
Use a fork to fluff. Serve warm.

✓ In a medium bowl, whisk eggs and cream together. Pour into a 4-cup round baking dish. Add cauliflower and mix, then top with Cheddar. Place dish into the air fryer basket. Adjust the temperature to 320°F and set the timer for 20 minutes.

✓ When completely cooked, eggs will be firm and cheese will be browned. Slice into four pieces.

✓ Slice avocado and divide evenly among pieces. Top

each piece with 2 tablespoons sour cream, sliced scallions, and crumbled bacon.

PER SERVING

Calories: 359

Protein: 19.5 G Fiber: 0.0 G

Net Carbohydrates: 1.1 G Fat: 27.6 G

Sodium: 325 Mg Carbohydrates: 1.1 G Sugar: 0.5 G

Loaded Cauliflower Breakfast Bake

Casseroles aren't just for dinnertime! This is the perfect option for busy weekday mornings, giving you lots of classic breakfast flavor and swapping in cauliflower where potatoes might usually be. Add a dash of hot sauce for some kick if you really want to wake up!

• HandsOn Time: 15 minutes • Cook Time: 20 minutes Serves 4

- 6 large eggs
- 1/4 cup heavy whipping cream
- 11/2 cups chopped cauliflower
- 1 cup shredded medium Cheddar cheese
- 1 medium avocado, peeled and pitted
- 8 tablespoons full-fat sour cream 2 scallions, sliced on the bias
- 12 slices sugar-free bacon, cooked and crumbled

    Directions

PER SERVING

Calories: 512 Protein: 27.1 G Fiber: 3.2 G
Net Carbohydrates: 4.3 G Fat: 38.3 G Sodium: 865 Mg Carbohydrates: 7.5 G Sugar: 2.3 G

Cinnamon Roll Sticks

With sweet and gooey cinnamon perfection, you'll have a rich start to your morning and guaranteed trouble sharing these Cinnamon Roll Sticks!

• HandsOn Time: 10 minutes • Cook Time: 7 minutes
Serves 4 (2 sticks per serving)

- 1 cup shredded mozzarella cheese
- 1 ounce full-fat cream cheese
- 1/3 cup blanched finely ground almond flour
- 1/2 teaspoon baking soda
- 1/2 cup granular erythritol, divided 1 teaspoon vanilla extract
- 1 large egg
- 2 tablespoons unsalted butter, melted
- 1/2 teaspoon ground cinnamon
- 3 tablespoons powdered erythritol
- 2 teaspoons unsweetened vanilla almond milk

Directions

✓ Place mozzarella in a large microwave-safe bowl and break cream cheese into small pieces and place into bowl. Microwave for 45 seconds.

✓ Stir in almond flour, baking soda, V4 cup granular erythritol, and vanilla. A soft dough should form. Microwave the mix for additional 15 seconds if it becomes too stiff.

✓ Mix egg into the dough, using your hands if necessary.

✓ Cut a piece of parchment to fit your air fryer basket. Press the dough into an 8" x 5" rectangle on the parchment and cut into eight (1") sticks.

✓ In a small bowl, mix butter, cinnamon, and remaining granular erythritol. Brush half the mixture over the top of the sticks and place them into the air fryer basket.

✓ Adjust the temperature to 400°F and set the timer for 7 minutes.

✓ Halfway through the cooking time, flip the sticks and brush with remaining butter mixture. When done, sticks should be crispy.

✓ To make glaze, whisk powdered erythritol and almond milk in a small bowl. Drizzle over cinnamon sticks. Serve warm.

PER SERVING

Calories: 233 Protein: 10.3 G Fiber: 1.2 G

Net Carbohydrates: 2.2 G Sugar Alcohol: 36.8 G Fat: 19.0 G Sodium: 378 Mg Carbohydrates: 40.2 G Sugar: 1.0 G

Breakfast Calzone

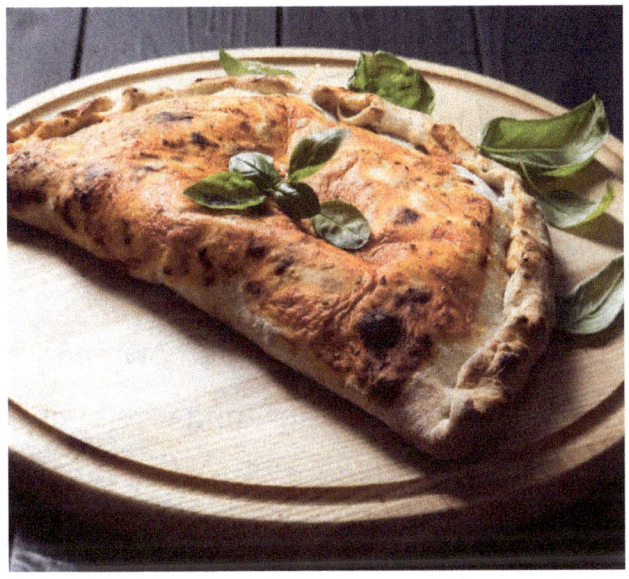

This is a great, and portable, way to start your morning! You can customize the filling with all of your favorites, freeze it the night before, and warm it up in your air fryer before taking it with you on your morning commute!

• HandsOn Time: 15 minutes • Cook Time: 15 minutes Serves 4

- 1 1/2 cups shredded mozzarella cheese
- 1/2 cup blanched finely ground almond flour

- 1 ounce full-fat cream cheese 1 large whole egg

- 4 large eggs, scrambled

- 1/2 pound cooked breakfast sausage,

- crumbled 8 tablespoons shredded mild Cheddar cheese

Directions

- ✓ In a large microwave-safe bowl, add mozzarella, almond flour, and cream cheese. Microwave for 1 minute. Stir until the mixture is smooth and forms a ball. Add the egg and stir until dough forms.

- ✓ Place dough between two sheets of parchment and roll out to V4" thickness. Cut the dough into four rectangles.

- ✓ Mix scrambled eggs and cooked sausage together in a large bowl. Divide the mixture evenly among each piece of dough, placing it on the lower half of the rectangle. Sprinkle each with 2 tablespoons Cheddar.

- ✓ Fold over the rectangle to cover the egg and meat mixture. Pinch, roll, or use a wet fork to close the edges completely.

- ✓ Cut a piece of parchment to fit your air fryer basket and place the calzones onto the parchment. Place parchment into the air fryer basket.

- ✓ Adjust the temperature to 380°F and set the timer for 15 minutes.

- ✓ Flip the calzones halfway through the cooking time. When done, calzones should be golden in color. Serve immediately.

PER SERVING

Calories: 560
Protein: 34.5 G
Fiber: 1.5 G
Net Carbohydrates: 4.2 G Fat: 41.7 G Sodium: 930 Mg Carbohydrates: 5.7 G Sugar: 2.1 G

Cauliflower Avocado Toast

Disappointed you can't keep up with the trend of avocado toast? Have no fear, this swap is a tasty, crunchy nutrient-rich breakfast that's full of healthy fats to help keep you full and focused throughout the day!

• HandsOn Time: 15 minutes • Cook Time: 8 minutes Serves 2 1 (12-ounce) steamer bag cauliflower 1 large egg

- 1/2 cup shredded mozzarella cheese
- 1 ripe medium avocado
- 1/2 teaspoon garlic powder
- 1/4 teaspoon ground black pepper

Directions

✓ Cook cauliflower according to package instructions. Remove from bag and place into cheesecloth or clean towel to remove excess moisture.

✓ Place cauliflower into a large bowl and mix in egg and mozzarella.

✓ Cut a piece of parchment to fit your air fryer basket.

✓ Separate the cauliflower mixture into two, and place it on the parchment in two mounds. Press out the cauliflower mounds into a 1/4"-thick rectangle.

✓ Place the parchment into the air fryer basket. Adjust the temperature to 400°F and set the timer for 8 minutes.

✓ Flip the cauliflower halfway through the cooking time. When the timer beeps, remove the parchment and allow the cauliflower to cool 5 minutes.

✓ Cut open the avocado and remove the pit. Scoop out the inside, place it in a medium bowl, and mash it with garlic powder and pepper. Spread onto the cauliflower. Serve immediately.

PER SERVING

Calories: 278
Protein: 14.1 G Fiber: 8.2 G
Net Carbohydrates: 7.7 G Fat: 15.6 G
Sodium: 267 Mg Carbohydrates: 15.9 G Sugar: 3.9 G

Sausage and Cheese Balls

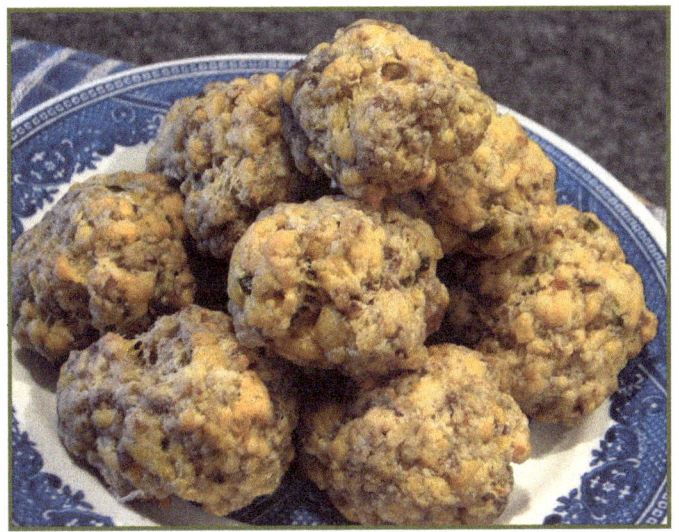

These breakfast-style meatballs make for a flavorful, protein- filled breakfast that you can make ahead of time, freeze, and pop into your air fryer when you're ready so your busy mornings are easy and delicious!

• HandsOn Time: 10 minutes • Cook Time: 12 minutes Yields 16 balls (4 per serving)

- 1 pound pork breakfast sausage
- 1/2 cup shredded Cheddar cheese

- 1 ounce full-fat cream cheese, softened 1 large egg

Directions

✓ Mix all ingredients in a large bowl. Form into sixteen (1") balls.

✓ Place the balls into the air fryer basket. Adjust the temperature to 400°F and set the timer for 12 minutes.

✓ Shake the basket two or three times during cooking. Sausage balls will be browned on the outside and have an internal temperature of at least 145°F when completely cooked. Serve warm.

PER SERVING

Calories: 424

Protein: 22.8 G Fiber: 0.0 G

Net Carbohydrates: 1.6 G Fat: 32.2 G

Sodium: 973 Mg Carbohydrates: 1.6 G Sugar: 1.4 G

FREEZER FRIENDLY!

These cheese balls are a great make-ahead item. If you want to freeze them, place cooked balls on a large cookie sheet and freeze for 1 hour. Then place in a freezer-safe storage bag.

Cheesy Bell Pepper Eggs

Bell peppers are a great source of vitamins A and C, two vitamins that are important for the strength of your immune system. This easy breakfast also gives you some protein from the ham and an extra boost of flavor from the onion. Altogether, you have a nutritious, well-rounded breakfast!

• HandsOn Time: 10 minutes • Cook Time: 15 minutes Serves 4

- 4 medium green bell peppers
- 3 ounces cooked ham, chopped
- 1/4 medium onion, peeled and chopped 8 large eggs
- 1 cup mild Cheddar cheese

Directions

✓ Cut the tops off each bell pepper. Remove the seeds and the white membranes with a small knife.

✓ Place ham and onion into each pepper.

✓ Crack 2 eggs into each pepper. Top with V4 cup cheese per pepper. Place into the air fryer basket.

✓ Adjust the temperature to 390°F and set the timer for 15 minutes.

✓ When fully cooked, peppers will be tender and eggs will be firm. Serve immediately.

PER SERVING

Calories: 314 protein: 24.9 g fiber: 1.7 g net carbs: 4.6 g fat: 18.6 g sodium: 621 mg sugar: 3.0 g

Spaghetti Squash Fritters

Squash is very quick to cook in the air fryer and has so many uses beyond just savory dinners. This dish is surprisingly flavorful and a breeze to make. Feel free to customize to your liking by adding your favorite filling items, such as mushrooms, chopped broccoli, or crumbled sausage.

• HandsOn Time: 15 minutes • Cook Time: 8 minutes

Serves 4

- 2 cups cooked spaghetti squash
- 2 tablespoons unsalted butter, softened
- 1 large egg
- 1/4 cup blanched finely ground almond flour
- 2 stalks green onion, sliced
- 1/2 teaspoon garlic powder
- 1 teaspoon dried parsley

Directions

✓ Remove excess moisture from the squash using a cheesecloth or kitchen towel.
✓ Mix all ingredients in a large bowl. Form into four patties.
✓ Cut a piece of parchment to fit your air fryer basket. Place each patty on the parchment and place into the air fryer basket.
✓ Adjust the temperature to 400°F and set the timer for 8 minutes. Flip the patties halfway through the cooking time. Serve warm.

Breakfast Egg Bowls

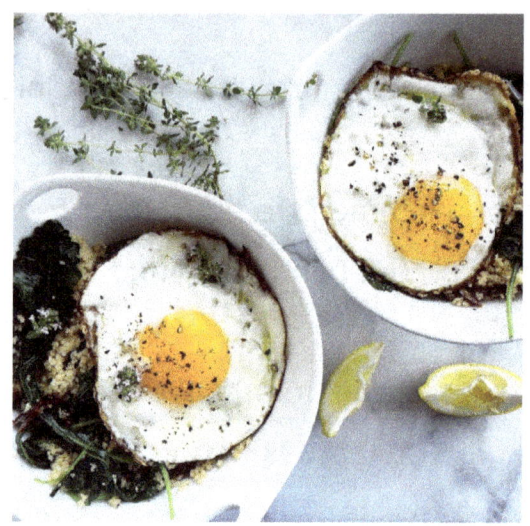

Preparation time: 10 minutes Cooking time: 20 minutes Servings: 4 Ingredients:

4 dinner rolls, tops cut off and insides scooped out 4 tablespoons heavy cream
4 eggs
4 tablespoons mixed chives and parsley

Salt and black pepper to the taste 4 tablespoons parmesan, grated

Directions

✓ Arrange dinner rolls on a baking sheet and crack an egg in each.

✓ Divide heavy cream, mixed herbs in each roll and season with salt and pepper.

✓ Sprinkle parmesan on top of your rolls, place them in your air fryer and cook at 350 degrees F for 20 minutes.

✓ Divide your bread bowls on plates and serve for breakfast. Enjoy!

Nutrition

calories 238, fat 4, fiber 7, carbs 14, protein 7

Delicious Breakfast Soufflé Preparation

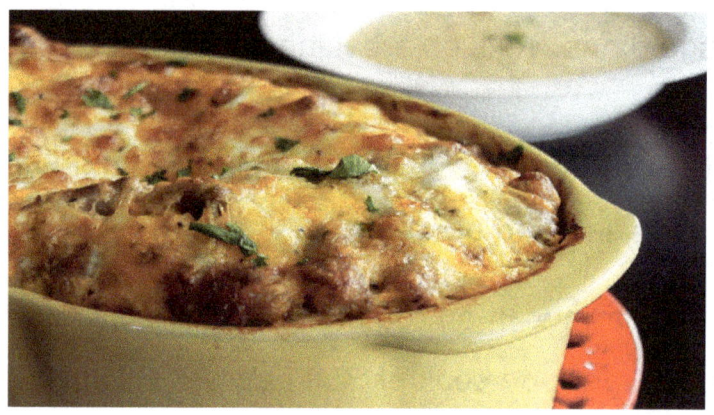

Preparation time: 10 minutes Cooking time: 8 minutes Servings: 4

Ingredients:

4 eggs, whisked

4 tablespoons heavy cream

A pinch of red chili pepper, crushed 2 tablespoons parsley, chopped

2 tablespoons chives, chopped

Salt and black pepper to the taste

Nutrition

calories 238, fat 4, fiber 7, carbs 14, protein 7

Directions

✓ In a bowl, mix eggs with salt, pepper, heavy cream, red chili pepper, parsley and chives, stir well and divide into 4 soufflé dishes.

✓ Arrange dishes in your air fryer and cook soufflés at 350 degrees F for 8 minutes.

✓ Serve them hot. Enjoy!

Nutrition

calories 300, fat 7, fiber 9, carbs 15, protein 6

Air Fried Sandwich

Time 10 minutes Cooking time: 6 minutes Servings: 2

Ingredients:

2 English muffins, halved
2 eggs
2 bacon strips
Salt and black pepper to the taste

Directions:

✓ Crack eggs in your air fryer, add bacon on top, cover and cook at 392 degrees F for 6 minutes.

✓ Heat up your English muffin halves in your microwave for a few seconds.

✓ Divide eggs on 2 halves, add bacon on top, season with salt and pepper, cover with the other 2 English muffins and serve for breakfast.

Enjoy!

Nutrition calories 261, fat 5, fiber 8, carbs 12, protein 4

Rustic Breakfast Preparation

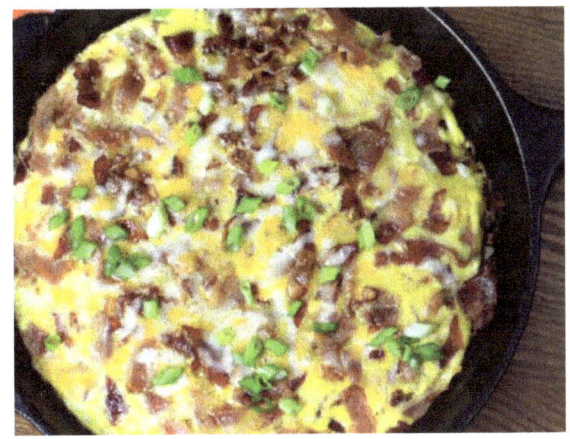

Time 10 minutes Cooking time: 13 minutes

Servings: 4

Ingredients

7 ounces baby spinach

8 chestnuts mushrooms, halved 8 tomatoes, halved

1 garlic clove, minced

4 chipolatas

4 bacon slices, chopped

Salt and black pepper to the taste 4 eggs

Cooking spray

Directions

✓ Grease a cooking pan with the oil and add tomatoes, garlic and mushrooms.

✓ Add bacon and chipolatas, also add spinach and crack eggs at the end.

✓ Season with salt and pepper, place pan in the cooking basket of your air fryer and cook for 13 minutes at 350 degrees F.

✓ Divide among plates and serve for breakfast. Enjoy!

Nutrition

calories 312, fat 6, fiber 8, carbs 15, protein 5

Egg Muffins Preparation

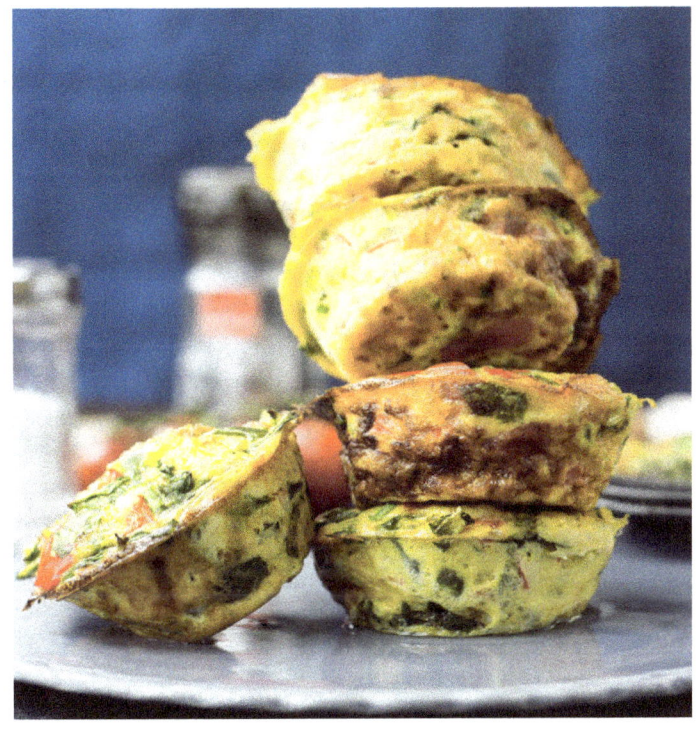

Time 10 minutes Cooking time: 15 minutes Servings: 4

Ingredients

1 egg
2 tablespoons olive oil
3 tablespoons milk
3.5 ounces white flour
1 tablespoon baking powder

2 ounces parmesan, grated

A splash of Worcestershire sauce

Directions

✓ In a bowl, mix egg with flour, oil, baking powder, milk, Worcestershire and parmesan, whisk well and divide into 4 silicon muffin cups.

✓ Arrange cups in your air fryer's cooking basket, cover and cook at 392, degrees F for 15 minutes. Serve warm for breakfast. Enjoy!

Nutrition

calories 251, fat 6, fiber 8, carbs 9, protein 3

Polenta Bites

Preparation time: 10 minutes Cooking time: 20 minutes Servings: 4

Ingredients

For the polenta:

1 tablespoon butter
1 cup cornmeal
3 cups water
Salt and black pepper to the taste

For the polenta bites:

2 tablespoons powdered sugar Cooking spray

Directions

√ In a pan, mix water with cornmeal, butter, salt and pepper, stir, bring to a boil over medium heat, cook for 10 minutes, take off heat, whisk one more time and keep in the fridge until it's cold.

√ Scoop 1 tablespoon of polenta, shape a ball and place on a working surface.

✓ Repeat with the rest of the polenta, arrange all the balls in the cooking basket of your air fryer, spray them with cooking spray, cover and cook at 380 degrees F for 8 minutes.

✓ Arrange polenta bites on plates, sprinkle sugar all over and serve for breakfast. Enjoy!

Nutrition

calories 231, fat 7, fiber 8, carbs 12, protein 4

Delicious Breakfast Potatoes

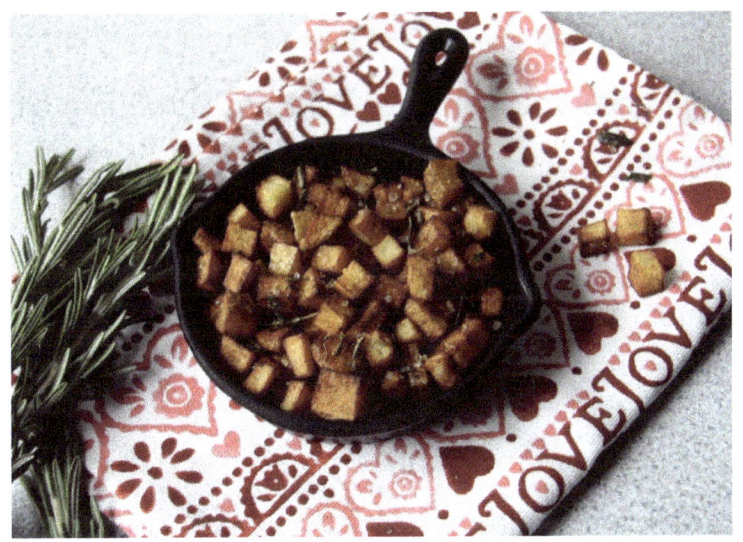

Preparation time: 10 minutes Cooking time: 35 minutes Servings: 4

Ingredients

2 tablespoons olive oil
3 potatoes, cubed
1 yellow onion, chopped
1 red bell pepper, chopped
Salt and black pepper to the taste 1 teaspoon garlic powder

1 teaspoon sweet paprika

1 teaspoon onion powder

Directions

✓ Grease your air fryer's basket with olive oil, add potatoes, toss and season with salt and pepper.

✓ Add onion, bell pepper, garlic powder, paprika and onion powder, toss well, cover and cook at 370 degrees F for 30 minutes.

✓ Divide potatoes mix on plates and serve for breakfast. Enjoy!

Nutrition

calories 214, fat 6, fiber 8, carbs 15, protein 4

Tasty Cinnamon Toast

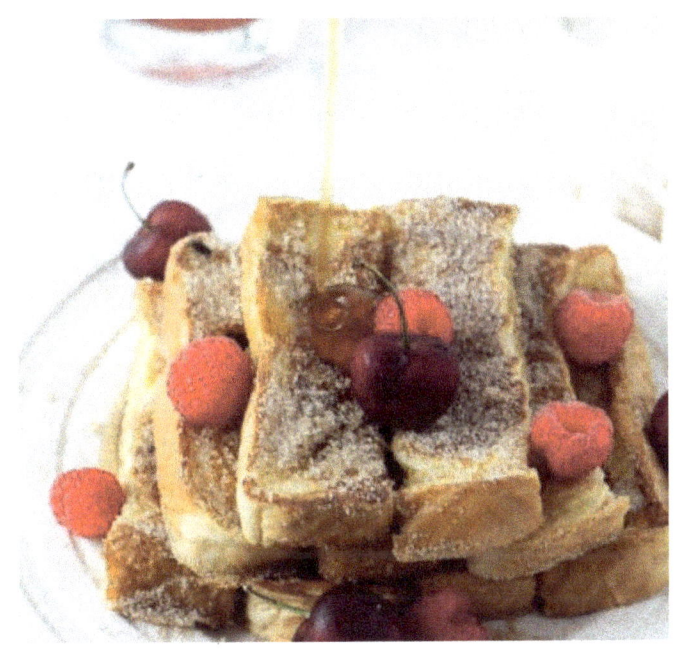

Preparation time: 10 minutes Cooking time: 5 minutes
Servings: 6

Ingredients

1 stick butter, soft
12 bread slices
1/2 cup brown sugar
1 and 1/2 teaspoon vanilla extract
1 and 1/2 teaspoon cinnamon powder

Directions

✓ In a bowl, mix soft butter with sugar, vanilla and cinnamon and whisk well.

✓ Spread this on bread slices, place them in your air fryer and cook at 400 degrees F for 5 minutes,

✓ Divide among plates and serve for breakfast. Enjoy!

Nutrition

calories 221, fat 4, fiber 7, carbs 12, protein 8

Delicious Potato Hash

Preparation time: 10 minutes Cooking time: 25 minutes Servings: 4

Ingredients

1 and 1/2 potatoes, cubed
1 yellow onion, chopped
2 teaspoons olive oil
1 green bell pepper, chopped Salt and black pepper to the taste 1/2 teaspoon thyme, dried 2 eggs

Directions

✓ Heat up your air fryer at 350 degrees F, add oil, heat it up, add onion, bell pepper, salt and pepper, stir and cook for 5 minutes.

✓ Add potatoes, thyme and eggs, stir, cover and cook at 360 degrees F for 20 minutes.

✓ Divide among plates and serve for breakfast. Enjoy!

Nutrition

calories 241, fat 4, fiber 7, carbs 12, protein 7

Sweet Breakfast Casserole

Preparation time: 10 minutes Cooking time: 30 minutes Servings: 4

Ingredients

3 tablespoons brown sugar

4 tablespoons butter

2 tablespoons white sugar

1/2 teaspoon cinnamon powder 1/2 cup flour

For the casserole:

2 eggs

2 tablespoons white sugar 2 and 1/2 cups white flour

1 teaspoon baking soda

1 teaspoon baking powder 2 eggs

1/2 cup milk

2 cups buttermilk

4 tablespoons butter

Zest from 1 lemon, grated 1 and 2/3 cup blueberries

Directions

√ In a bowl, mix eggs with 2 tablespoons white sugar, 2 and 1/2 cups white flour, baking powder, baking soda, 2 eggs, milk, buttermilk, 4 tablespoons butter, lemon zest and blueberries, stir and pour into a pan that fits your air fryer.

√ In another bowls, mix 3 tablespoons brown sugar with 2 tablespoons white sugar, 4 tablespoons butter, 1/2 cup flour and cinnamon, stir until you obtain a crumble and spread over blueberries mix.

√ Place in preheated air fryer and bake at 300 degrees F for 30 minutes.

√ Divide among plates and serve for breakfast. Enjoy!

Nutrition: calories 214, fat 5, fiber 8, carbs 12, protein 5

Eggs Casserole

Preparation time: 10 minutes Cooking time: 25 minutes Servings: 6 Ingredients:

1 pound turkey, ground 1 tablespoon olive oil 1/2 teaspoon chili powder 12 eggs

1 sweet potato, cubed
1 cup baby spinach
Salt and black pepper to the taste 2 tomatoes, chopped for serving

Directions

✓ In a bowl, mix eggs with salt, pepper, chili powder, potato, spinach, turkey and sweet potato and whisk well.

✓ Heat up your air fryer at 350 degrees F, add oil and heat it up.

✓ Add eggs mix, spread into your air fryer, cover and cook for 25 minutes.

✓ Divide among plates and serve for breakfast. Enjoy!

Nutrition: calories 300, fat 5, fiber 8, carbs 13, protein 6

Sausage, Eggs and Cheese Mix

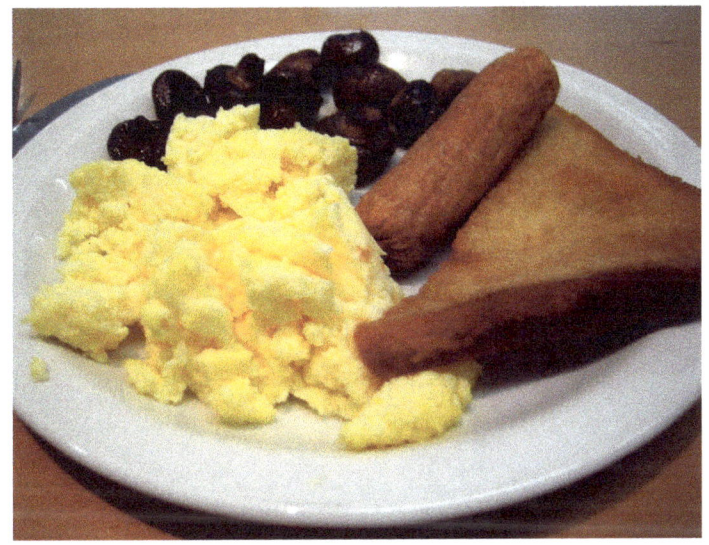

Preparation time: 10 minutes Cooking time: 20 minutes Servings: 4

Ingredients:

10 ounces sausages, cooked and crumbled 1 cup cheddar cheese, shredded

1 cup mozzarella cheese, shredded

8 eggs, whisked

1 cup milk

Salt and black pepper to the taste Cooking spray

Directions

✓ In a bowl, mix sausages with cheese, mozzarella, eggs, milk, salt and pepper and whisk well.

✓ Heat up your air fryer at 380 degrees F, spray cooking oil, add eggs and sausage mix and cook for 20 minutes.

✓ Divide among plates and serve. Enjoy!

Nutrition: calories 320, fat 6, fiber 8, carbs 12, protein 5

Cheese Air Fried Bake

Preparation time: 10 minutes Cooking time: 20 minutes Servings: 4

4 bacon slices, cooked and crumbled
2 cups milk
2 and 1/2 cups cheddar cheese, shredded
1 pound breakfast sausage, casings removed and chopped 2 eggs
1/2 teaspoon onion powder Salt and black pepper to the taste
3 tablespoons parsley, chopped, Cooking spray

Directions

√ In a bowl, mix eggs with milk, cheese, onion powder, salt, pepper and parsley and whisk well.

√ Grease your air fryer with cooking spray, heat it up at 320 degrees F and add bacon and sausage.

√ Add eggs mix, spread and cook for 20 minutes.

√ Divide among plates and serve. Enjoy!

Nutrition calories 214, fat 5, fiber 8, carbs 12, protein 12

Biscuits Casserole

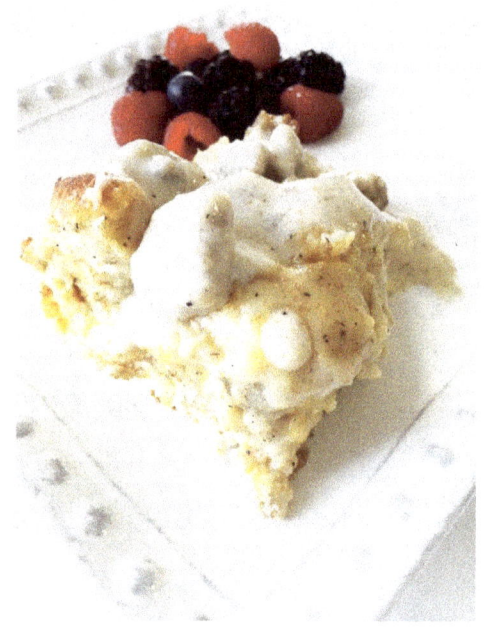

Preparation time: 10 minutes Cooking time: 15 minutes Servings: 8

Ingredients

12 ounces biscuits, quartered
3 tablespoons flour
1/2 pound sausage, chopped
A pinch of salt and black pepper 2 and 1/2 cups milk
Cooking spray

Directions

✓ Grease your air fryer with cooking spray and heat it over 350 degrees F.

✓ Add biscuits on the bottom and mix with sausage. Add flour, milk, salt and pepper, toss a bit and cook for 15 minutes.

✓ Divide among plates and serve for breakfast. Enjoy!

Nutrition

calories 321, fat 4, fiber 7, carbs 12, protein 5

Turkey Burrito

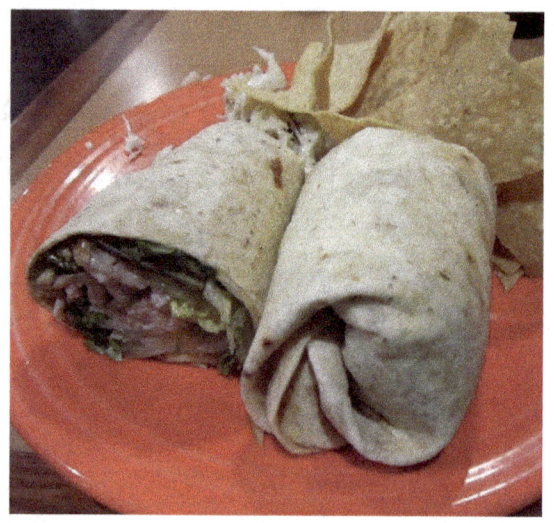

Preparation time: 10 minutes Cooking time: 10 minutes Servings: 2

Ingredients

4 slices turkey breast already cooked
1/2 red bell pepper, sliced
2 eggs
1 small avocado, peeled, pitted and sliced 2 tablespoons salsa

Salt and black pepper to the taste 1/8 cup mozzarella cheese, grated Tortillas for serving

Directions

√ In a bowl, whisk eggs with salt and pepper to the taste, pour them in a pan and place it in the air fryer's basket.

√ Cook at 400 degrees F for 5 minutes, take pan out of the fryer and transfer eggs to a plate.

√ Arrange tortillas on a working surface, divide eggs on them, also divide turkey meat, bell pepper, cheese, salsa and avocado.

√ Roll your burritos and place them in your air fryer after you've lined it with some tin foil.

√ Heat up the burritos at 300 degrees F for 3 minutes, divide them on plates and serve. Enjoy!

Nutrition

calories 349, fat 23, fiber 11, carbs 20, protein 21

Tofu Scramble

Preparation time: 5 minutes Cooking time: 30 minutes Servings: 4

Ingredients

2 tablespoons soy sauce
1 tofu block, cubed
1 teaspoon turmeric, ground
2 tablespoons extra virgin olive oil 4 cups broccoli florets
1/2 teaspoon onion powder
1/2 teaspoon garlic powder
2 and 1/2 cup red potatoes, cubed
1/2 cup yellow onion, chopped
Salt and black pepper to the taste

Directions

√ Mix tofu with 1 tablespoon oil, salt, pepper, soy sauce, garlic powder, onion powder, turmeric and onion in a bowl, stir and leave aside.

√ In a separate bowl, combine potatoes with the rest of the oil, a pinch of salt and pepper and toss to coat.

✓ Put potatoes in your air fryer at 350 degrees F and bake for 15 minutes, shaking once.

✓ Add tofu and its marinade to your air fryer and bake for 15 minutes.

✓ Add broccoli to the fryer and cook everything for 5 minutes more. Serve right away. Enjoy!

Nutrition

calories 140, fat 4, fiber 3, carbs 10, protein 14

Oatmeal Casserole

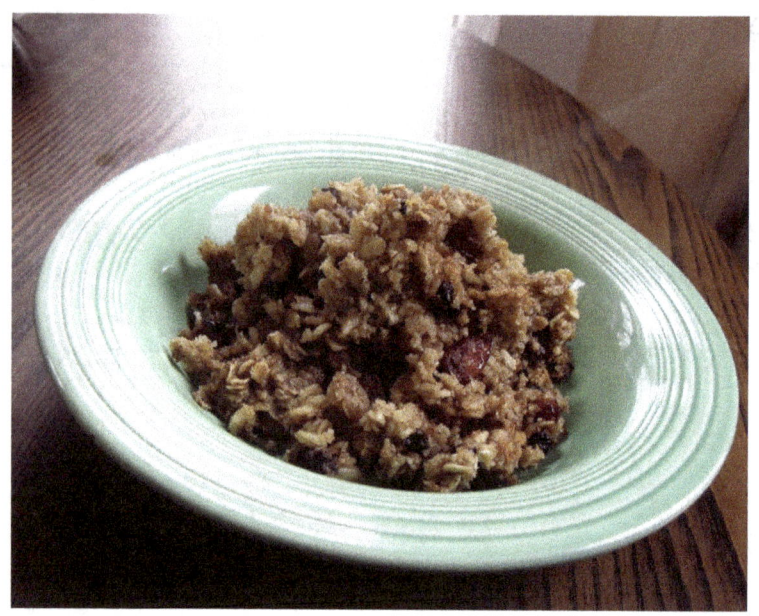

Preparation time: 10 minutes Cooking time: 20 minutes Servings: 8

Ingredients

2 cups rolled oats

1 teaspoon baking powder 1/3 cup brown sugar

1 teaspoon cinnamon powder 1/2 cup chocolate chips

2/3 cup blueberries

1 banana, peeled and mashed 2 cups milk

1 eggs

2 tablespoons butter

1 teaspoon vanilla extract Cooking spray

Directions

✓ In a bowl, mix sugar with baking powder, cinnamon, chocolate chips, blueberries and banana and stir.

✓ In a separate bowl, mix eggs with vanilla extract and butter and stir.

✓ Heat up your air fryer at 320 degrees F, grease with cooking spray and add oats on the bottom.

✓ Add cinnamon mix and eggs mix, toss and cook for 20 minutes.

✓ Stir one more time, divide into bowls and serve for breakfast. Enjoy!

Nutrition

calories 300, fat 4, fiber 7, carbs 12, protein 10

Ham Breakfast

Preparation time: 10 minutes Cooking time: 15 minutes Servings: 6

Ingredients

6 cups French bread, cubed
4 ounces green chilies, chopped 10 ounces ham, cubed
4 ounces cheddar cheese, shredded 2 cups milk
5 eggs
1 tablespoon mustard
Salt and black pepper to the taste Cooking spray

Directions

√ Heat up your air fryer at 350 degrees F and grease it with cooking spray. In a bowl, mix eggs with milk, cheese, mustard, salt and pepper and stir.

√ Add bread cubes in your air fryer and mix with chilies and ham. Add eggs mix, spread and cook for 15 minutes.

✓ Divide among plates and serve. Enjoy!

Nutrition

calories 200, fat 5, fiber 6, carbs 12, protein 14

Tomato and Bacon Breakfast

Preparation time: 10 minutes Cooking time: 30 minutes Servings: 6

Ingredients

1 pound white bread, cubed

1 pound smoked bacon, cooked and chopped 1/4 cup olive oil

1 yellow onion, chopped

28 ounces canned tomatoes, chopped 1/2 teaspoon red pepper, crushed

1/2 pound cheddar, shredded

2 tablespoons chives, chopped

1/2 pound Monterey jack, shredded

2 tablespoons stock

Salt and black pepper to the taste

8 eggs, whisked

Directions

✓ Add the oil to your air fryer and heat it up at 350 degrees F.

✓ Add bread, bacon, onion, tomatoes, red pepper and stock and stir.

✓ Add eggs, cheddar and Monterey jack and cook everything for 20 minutes.

✓ Divide among plates, sprinkle chives and serve. Enjoy!

Nutrition

calories 231, fat 5, fiber 7, carbs 12, protein 4

Tasty Hash

Preparation time: 10 minutes Cooking time: 15 minutes Servings: 6

Ingredients

16 ounces hash browns
1/4 cup olive oil
1/2 teaspoon paprika
1/2 teaspoon garlic powder
Salt and black pepper to the taste 1 egg, whisked

2 tablespoon chives, chopped 1 cup cheddar, shredded

Directions

✓ Add oil to your air fryer, heat it up at 350 degrees F and add hash browns.

✓ Also add paprika, garlic powder, salt, pepper and egg, toss and cook for 15 minutes.

✓ Add cheddar and chives, toss, divide among plates and serve. Enjoy!

Nutrition calories 213, fat 7, fiber 8, carbs 12, protein 4

Creamy Hash Browns

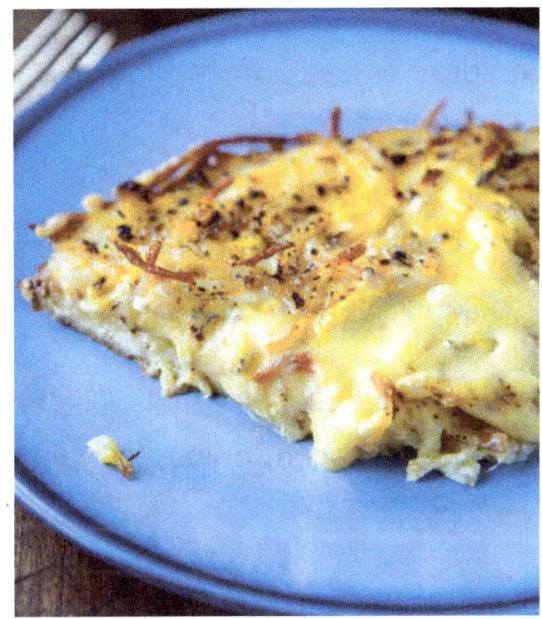

Preparation time: 10 minutes Cooking time: 20 minutes Servings: 6

Ingredients

2 pounds hash browns

1 cup whole milk

8 bacon slices, chopped

9 ounces cream cheese

1 yellow onion, chopped

1 cup cheddar cheese, shredded 6 green onions, chopped

Salt and black pepper to the taste 6 eggs
Cooking spray

Directions

✓ Heat up your air fryer at 350 degrees F and grease it with cooking spray.

✓ In a bowl, mix eggs with milk, cream cheese, cheddar cheese, bacon, onion, salt and pepper and whisk well.

✓ Add hash browns to your air fryer, add eggs mix over them and cook for 20 minutes.

✓ Divide among plates and serve. Enjoy!

Nutrition

calories 261, fat 6, fiber 9, carbs 8, protein 12

Blackberry French Toast

Preparation time: 10 minutes Cooking time: 20 minutes Servings: 6

Ingredients

1 cup blackberry jam, warm 12 ounces bread loaf, cubed
8 ounces cream cheese, cubed 4 eggs
1 teaspoon cinnamon powder 2 cups half and half
1/2 cup brown sugar
1 teaspoon vanilla extract Cooking spray

Directions

✓ Grease your air fryer with cooking spray and heat it up at 300 degrees F.

✓ Add blueberry jam on the bottom, layer half of the bread cubes, then add cream cheese and top with the rest of the bread.

✓ In a bowl, mix eggs with half and half, cinnamon, sugar and vanilla, whisk well and add over bread mix.

✓ Cook for 20 minutes, divide among plates and serve for breakfast. Enjoy!

Nutrition

calories 215, fat 6, fiber 9, carbs 16, protein 6

Smoked Sausage Breakfast Mix

Preparation time: 10 minutes Cooking time: 30 minutes Servings: 4

Ingredients

1 and 1/2 pounds smoked sausage, chopped and browned A pinch of salt and black pepper

1 and 1/2 cups grits
4 and 1/2 cups water
16 ounces cheddar cheese, shredded 1 cup milk
1/4 teaspoon garlic powder
1 and 1/2 teaspoons thyme, chopped Cooking spray
4 eggs, whisked

Directions

√ Put the water in a pot, bring to a boil over medium heat, add grits, stir, cover, cook for 5 minutes and take off heat.

√ Add cheese, stir until it melts and mix with milk, thyme, salt, pepper, garlic powder and eggs and whisk really well.

✓ Heat up your air fryer at 300 degrees F, grease with cooking spray and add browned sausage.

✓ Add grits mix, spread and cook for 25 minutes.

✓ Divide among plates and serve for breakfast. Enjoy!

Nutrition

calories 321, fat 6, fiber 7, carbs 17, protein 4

Delicious Potato Frittata

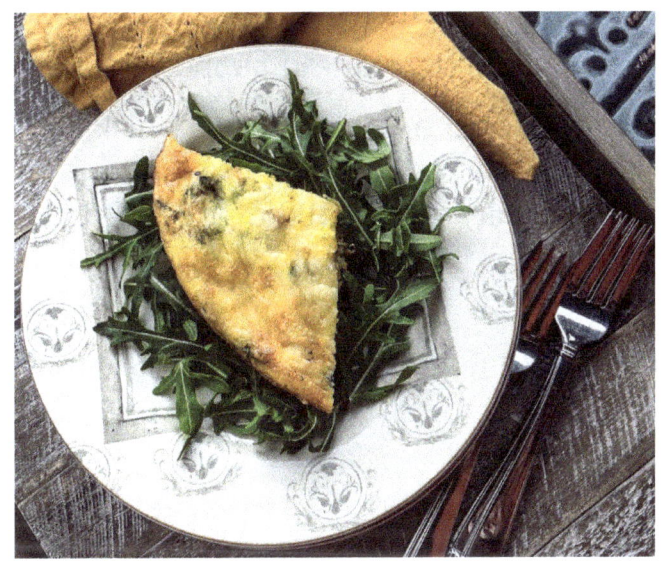

Preparation time: 10 minutes Cooking time: 20 minutes Servings: 6

Ingredients

6 ounces jarred roasted red bell peppers, chopped 12 eggs, whisked
1/2 cup parmesan, grated
3 garlic cloves, minced

2 tablespoons parsley, chopped Salt and black pepper to the taste 2 tablespoons chives, chopped 16 potato wedges

6 tablespoons ricotta cheese Cooking spray

Directions

✓ In a bowl, mix eggs with red peppers, garlic, parsley, salt, pepper and ricotta and whisk well.

✓ Heat up your air fryer at 300 degrees F and grease it with cooking spray.

✓ Add half of the potato wedges on the bottom and sprinkle half of the parmesan all over.

✓ Add half of the egg mix, add the rest of the potatoes and the rest of the parmesan.

✓ Add the rest of the eggs mix, sprinkle chives and cook for 20 minutes.

✓ Divide among plates and serve for breakfast. Enjoy!

Nutrition

calories 312, fat 6, fiber 9, carbs 16, protein 5

Asparagus Frittata

Preparation time: 10 minutes Cooking time: 5 minutes Servings: 2

Ingredients

4 eggs, whisked
2 tablespoons parmesan, grated 4 tablespoons milk
Salt and black pepper to the taste 10 asparagus tips, steamed Cooking spray

Directions

√ In a bowl, mix eggs with parmesan, milk, salt and pepper and whisk well.

√ Heat up your air fryer at 400 degrees F and grease with cooking spray.

√ Add asparagus, add eggs mix, toss a bit and cook for 5 minutes.

√ Divide frittata on plates and serve for breakfast. Enjoy!

Nutrition calories 312, fat 5, fiber 8, carbs 14, protein 2

Special Corn Flakes Breakfast Casserole

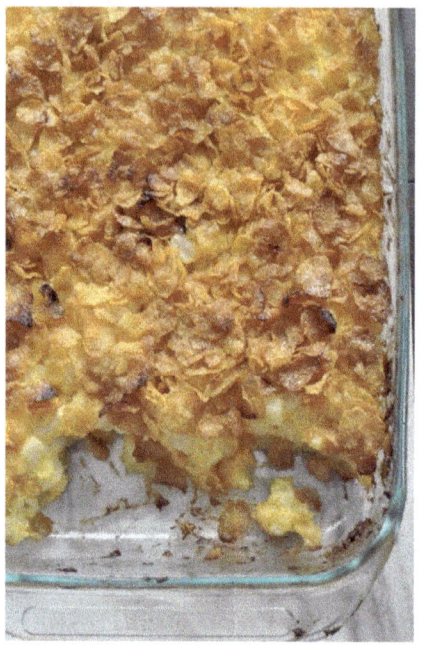

Preparation time: 10 minutes Cooking time: 8 minutes Servings: 5

Ingredients

1/3 cup milk

3 teaspoons sugar

2 eggs, whisked

1/4 teaspoon nutmeg, ground

1/4 cup blueberries

4 tablespoons cream cheese, whipped 1 and 1/2 cups

corn flakes, crumbled

5 bread slices

Directions

√ In a bowl, mix eggs with sugar, nutmeg and milk and whisk well. In another bowl, mix cream cheese with blueberries and whisk well.

√ Put corn flakes in a third bowl.
Spread blueberry mix on each bread slice, then dip in eggs mix and dredge in corn flakes at the end.

√ Place bread in your air fryer's basket, heat up at 400 degrees F and bake for 8 minutes.

√ Divide among plates and serve for breakfast. Enjoy!

Nutrition

calories 300, fat 5, fiber 7, carbs 16, protein 4

Ham Breakfast Pie

Preparation time: 10 minutes Cooking time: 25 minutes Servings: 6

Ingredients

16 ounces crescent rolls dough 2 eggs, whisked
2 cups cheddar cheese, grated
1 tablespoon parmesan, grated, 2 cups ham, cooked and chopped Salt and black pepper to the taste
Cooking spray

Directions

√ Grease your air fryer's pan with cooking spray and press half of the crescent rolls dough on the bottom.

√ In a bowl, mix eggs with cheddar cheese, parmesan, salt and pepper, whisk well and add over dough.

√ Spread ham, cut the rest of the crescent rolls dough in strips, arrange them over ham and cook at 300 degrees F for 25 minutes.

√ Slice pie and serve for breakfast. Enjoy!

Nutrition calories 400, fat 27, fiber 7, carbs 22, protein 16

Breakfast Veggie Mix

Preparation time: 10 minutes Cooking time: 25 minutes Servings: 6

Ingredients

1 yellow onion, sliced
1 red bell pepper, chopped
1 gold potato, chopped
2 tablespoons olive oil
8 ounces brie, trimmed and cubed 12 ounces sourdough bread, cubed 4 ounces parmesan, grated
8 eggs
2 tablespoons mustard
3 cups milk
Salt and black pepper to the taste

Directions

√ Heat up your air fryer at 350 degrees F, add oil, onion, potato and bell pepper and cook for 5 minutes.

√ In a bowl, mix eggs with milk, salt, pepper and mustard and whisk well.

√ Add bread and brie to your air fryer, add half of the eggs mix and add half of the parmesan as well.

✓ Add the rest of the bread and parmesan, toss just a little bit and cook for 20 minutes.

✓ Divide among plates and serve for breakfast. Enjoy!

Nutrition

calories 231, fat 5, fiber 10, carbs 20, protein 12

CPSIA information can be obtained
at www.ICGtesting.com
Printed in the USA
LVHW050323190421
684849LV00015B/814